How I Quit Snoring In One Night

Without Any Medications, Devices or Surgery

Julie G. Niehoff

DEDICATION

For CJ. Thanks for all the verve, babe.

CONTENTS

ACKNOWLEDGMENTS

Thank you to my husband CJ for enduring so many nights of lost sleep and 20+ years of deep love and great verve. Much appreciation to Jade and Calen for loving me enough to laugh about sleeping with headphones on when we had to share hotel rooms and for never telling me how bad it really was. And lots of love to little Gracie for being able to curl up and sleep right next to me anytime, no matter how loud I was snoring.

I also want to say thank you to the following people for continued love and support and for the various roles each has played in this journey to a good night's sleep. They are not listed in any particular order. Thank you to to Dan, Andy and Sonny Meunchow, Mark Chesterfield, Melanie & Derek Allen and Jason Vare, Bill Weir, John Castle, Mike, Jill and Laura Slaughter, Kate Tolliver and Annette Hawkins, my late grandparents, Gigi and Papa, John and Scott Larkin and my Mom & Dad

1 INTRODUCTION

I have been snoring since my first pregnancy in 1997. It's not pretty, especially as a woman. And while it did get both a little better and a little worse as my weight fluctuated up and down over time, nothing I tried seemed to do the trick.

My husband of 20+ years also snores sometimes, so it wasn't really that big of a deal at first. But somewhere around 2007, at the age of 40 and in the middle of another pregnancy, my snoring began to get worse.

I tried over the counter remedies, went to see medical doctors and even snoring specialists. I'll get more into what they told me in a bit. But around 2am in a very quiet hotel room in Lucerne, Switzerland in the fall of 2014, I finally figured out a way to stop my snoring.

This very short book will explain how I did it. I hope very much that it will help you – even if you do not have the same exact issues that I have, you may at least find a path to figuring out your own solution for snoring.

Happily, I have been able to get a nice, long, quiet night's sleep – as has my husband – every night since.

It is important that I state clearly that I am not a doctor, nor am I a medical professional. This book is not intended to provide medical advice. It is a story of my experiences with snoring and how I was able to stop. But after so many years of trying – and failing – to find a solution, I am compelled to share the very simple one that helped me.

2 EPIC SNORING IS NOT LIKE REGULAR SNORING

If you have an epic snore, then you already know it. Others have told you.

My husband snores, but it's that fairly common, every-once-in-a-while kind of snoring that I actually like and find comforting, knowing that he is there next to me. I used to snore like that and I'm told it was… well, it was kind of cute. Not actually cute, but kind of.

I think that assessment from a loved one came in retrospect, meaning AFTER everyone in the family had heard what a real snoring problem sounds like. My snoring, at its worst, could be heard across the entire house. I don't know how I slept through it. Apparently others could not.

My husband started having trouble sleeping next to me. Not good. We never actually switched to separate bedrooms, but it was coming to that soon if I hadn't stumbled onto my remedy.

I used to wake up and my husband would have his head at the foot of the bed and his feet would be where the pillows are. He would say it was because he was watching TV – which I do believe was true, at least at first, because the TV is across the room from the foot of our bed.

I am pretty sure he was shifting his position so that he could hear the TV over my snoring if I fell asleep first. But eventually, he just started staying in that position, sleeping there even after he was ready to go to sleep.

When we would have company staying over – which is pretty often – they would laugh with me in the kitchen over coffee and tell me that they heard my husband snoring all the way across the house in the middle of the night. Depending on my relationship with them, I would (usually) admit that it was more likely me that they heard. This admission never failed to produce some reaction of disbelief.

When I travel for work with other co-workers, I would always worry that one of them would be placed in the room next to mine, certain that I would be "outed" as an epic snorer by having terrible reverberations through the walls of the Embassy Suites. My defense mechanism for this was to come right out and ask what room people were in and when it was a friend, to say (yes, out loud) that I didn't want them to hear me snore. It was the very same kind of thing that a chubby kid does in school to poke fun at themselves before others could.

I could hear myself saying the words. And something in me knew this little game was a bad sign. But I didn't know how to fix it, so I kept going with what I had to work with.

3 JUMPING THROUGH HOOPS

As my snoring got worse and I found myself avoiding the need to sleep at other people's homes, staying awake as late as I could to make sure my husband was able to get some sleep before I ruined it with my crazy freight train, and really – when I realized I was considering sleeping in a different room from him because of this issue, I started to seek professional help.

I shouldn't have taken that long but denial is in my DNA and I just kept putting it off. If my sweet husband said that his lack of sleep wasn't all about my snoring, I chose to see that as confirmation that my snoring wasn't all that bad.

Never mind that he is a really nice guy who just doesn't want to make his wife feel like a troll. Or that I had begun waking up in the morning to find him with a wall of pillows encasing his head in a sort of goose down tomb, even when he was flipped around with his feet at the pillow end and his head six feet away from mine.

I had to find a solution. If for no other reason than to keep my husband from suffocating himself.

As humans living in these times, what do we do when we need solutions? We Google it. I googled snoring solutions, snoring problem, snoring causes, how to stop snoring – you name it, I googled it.

I found all kinds of remedies and devices that promised to stop my snoring. On reading the reviews, I wasn't very hopeful. But I should point out that I didn't order any. I did buy those strips that go on your nose. Didn't help me. They might help some people, but not me.

I tried throat sprays. Those didn't help me. I tried tying a scarf around my head. Looked stupid and still, no help.

I talked to my sister-in-law about her machine that helps pump oxygen into your airway while you sleep. I made an appointment to see a doctor and thought I would consider a sleep study to see about one of those machines.

But I also took a nap using hers to see what it was like. I know that these machines really help people and if your doctor tells you to use one, you should. I did not have a doctor tell me to use one. So I didn't. It wasn't what I would call a pleasant experience for me. She, however, found great relief for her sleep apnea and credits that device with a whole new life of real rest and better health down the line.

I am grateful that I do not have sleep apnea. That just wasn't my path. But I still needed a solution.

4 DOCTOR VISITS

I did go to the doctor. Several of them.

I talked to my regular MD about the problem and she suggested I see an ear, nose and throat specialist. So I made an appointment.

In the meantime, I also saw my endocrinologist. Side note – I have Hashimoto's Thyroiditis, an auto-immune disease that is related to my thyroid. As a result of this condition, I do have an enlarged thyroid (a butterfly-shaped gland in the throat).

I brought up my snoring with my endocrinologist because I thought that my disease might be contributing to my battle with snoring. She said it was possible and ordered an ultrasound to take a closer look. That turned up no real evidence and we continue to treat my thyroid but it didn't help with my snoring.

In the meantime, I also found; while again searching for an answer online, a medical practice near my home that actually has the word snoring in their name. I will not specifically name any of my doctors because they all gave me good care and I don't want to give the impression that they did not serve me or my health concerns in a professional and caring manner. They were all very kind and attentive and wonderful.

So here's what happened. I went to see the ear, nose and throat doctor and was told that I could have surgery to make the roof of my mouth and/or the back of my throat more stiff and therefore unable to "rattle" in snoring. I didn't really want to have surgery. A friend had already told me that she had this same surgery, as did her husband, and that it worked for a few months and then they were both right back to snoring. In separate rooms.

At the practice with snoring in the name, I had a really interesting experience. That doctor did an MRI of my head and I got some really cool images of my curly nasal passages. She also put a tiny camera up my nose and down my throat.

With those images, she showed me how one of my nasal passages is completely blocked. She also showed me where I had actually created a new sinus cavity inside my nasal passages. She pointed out that my regular sinuses were considered to be extremely small and then she told me that none of that was likely to be causing my epic snoring.

She did prescribe me a nasal spray and then before I left she said that she noticed my enlarged thyroid and asked if I would like to have her remove it.

I told her that I was working with an endocrinologist on my Hashimoto's and that we were not really discussing surgery at this time. I also asked her if having it removed would help my snoring and she said it wasn't likely but that she would be willing to take it out for me anytime if I decided that I wanted to do that. Okay. Good to know.

Here is something great that came out of that visit. For the next two nights, my husband reported that while I was still snoring, it was quite a bit softer than usual. Still louder than your average grizzly bear but not like it had been in recent weeks.

I filled the nasal spray prescription thinking that maybe it was the same thing she had sprayed in my nose and throat to get the tiny camera in. We were hopeful that this spray was part of a solution since I was a little quieter after the camera visit.

But, the prescription did not have the same effect. I even called to ask if it was the same as what she sprayed into my nose in her office, and learned it wasn't. I tried to get some of that but she did not give it to me and I still do not know what it was.

The good news was that it was possible to at least be quieter. Knowing this, I forged ahead with a little hope. Sometimes, that's what you need to keep going toward a bigger solution. I was grateful for at least that.

5 A FATEFUL TRIP TO SWITZERLAND

In the Fall of 2014, my husband and I went on a trip to the UK and Switzerland. I had some work in London and he had scheduled a short tour – he is a blues musician – in Lucerne and other cities along the way. I was excited to go, but also a little worried that I still hadn't solved my snoring issues.

What was going to happen if I was snoring and my husband was trapped for two weeks in hotel rooms, unable to get away from me?

We packed up and set off for this adventure together. The 3rd night, there was a moment where he woke me up from a deep sleep/snore and he asked me to turn over. He doesn't usually do that. I figured this meant that it was pretty bad.

I tried to stay awake but it wasn't working. He didn't sleep much. I felt terrible about it. Apart from this, our trip was really perfect. My stupid snoring was the dark spot on an otherwise wonderful time.

The second half of our trip was in Switzerland. While in London, we'd stayed in a familiar hotel, a chain with a name you would recognize. But in Switzerland, my husband's tour manager had set up the accommodations. Our hotel was very clean and nice, but also very … what is the word? Sparse.

There was no TV, no telephone and no free internet or Wi-Fi. But we didn't really care about any of that. Who wanted to watch TV? We were surrounded by postcard-perfect scenery and amazing people, food, drink and sites to explore. OK, we did care a little about the internet access.

The real and honestly only issue with the hotel room was that there was no carpeting and the walls were paper thin. Consider an epic snore in a room with nothing to dampen the sound. In a room with no carpet, all sounds reverberate onto all surfaces like an amplifier. Now add paper thin walls.

I have no idea how many people were kept awake by my snoring. I do know of one for sure. My husband.

Again, he woke me up. And not quite as gently as the last time. I was a little stuffed up but the lack of sound-absorbing carpet together with my epic snore had him looking like that guy in *A Clockwork Orange* who is tortured by having his eyes propped open by toothpicks. Even if you haven't seen the movie, you get the picture.

He was so, so tired and unable to get away from me the way he might at home. In Austin, he might get up and walk around, sleep on the couch in the family room for a bit, walk outside and play some guitar on the back porch, whatever – there were options to get away from the noise.

But at that moment, in that room, with that hard wood floor and no extra pillow to wrap around his head, he was understandably at a breaking point.

I think it's only fair to say that he was still nice about it. Somehow. But I could see on his face that it wasn't ok to just deal with it. I figured that when we got home, we would probably be sleeping in separate rooms. And I felt really bad. I sat up and told him I would stay up so he could sleep.

He didn't argue with me. He rolled over and went to sleep. I sat in the dark for a while and decided to turn on my laptop. We had purchased an hour of internet access at the front desk in case I wanted to video chat with my kiddos. I had around 20 minutes left on that, so I decided to look one last time for a solution to my snoring.

6 THE BIG MOMENT

I clicked on my browser, typed in google.com and started my all too familiar search for a solution. I did notice that I was on the Swiss version of the site, but it had an English option so I didn't give it much thought.

But on my first search, I noticed that there were different options for information than what always came up first for me back home.

In the US when I google this issue, I come to hundreds of sites about devices and medical surgeries to stop snoring. In Switzerland, I landed quickly on a site that asked "Are you a tongue snorer?"

That was completely new to me. Four doctors, nasal strips, sprays, scarves and hours of googling and reading and nobody had ever posed this question.

The site said to stick out your tongue as far as you could and try to replicate your snoring sound. If, with your tongue out, your snore was significantly softer, then you are a tongue snorer.

Ladies and gentlemen, as it turns out, I am a tongue snorer. Sitting in my hotel room with no carpet and with my husband finally sleeping, sticking out my tongue. It was a huge moment. Bigger than I realized at that moment.

And then, the Internet stopped on me. I had no more time online. I couldn't go down and buy more time either. The front desk was closed. Actually closed. It's not a Hilton in Dallas. Feel me?

I turned off the computer and sat on the bed, sticking my tongue out and trying to make myself snore. All while trying not to make a lot of noise so that my husband could sleep.

After an hour or so, and once he was doing his regular people snoring so I knew he was really asleep, I decided to just lie down for a bit. And then as I lay there, I stuck my tongue out as far as I could and held it between two fingers. I felt like an idiot but I figured it couldn't hurt to try.

I completely relaxed my throat and wasn't snoring. I was breathing through my nose. I did get up and spray some simple saline spray into my nostrils, to try and make sure my nose wouldn't close up on me if I fell asleep that way. And then I lay back down, held my tongue in my fingertips and went to sleep.

In the morning, I woke up and my husband was still asleep. I didn't say anything about it because, well, what am I going to say? "I think I didn't snore last night because I slept with my tongue sticking out!" He didn't wake up so I was happy. Still not really celebration worthy – at least not yet.

The next night, before we went to sleep, I sprayed the simple nasal spray and turned away from my husband hoping he would not notice that I was holding my tongue with my fingertips. I pulled my blanket up around my chin to help hide it as well. And I went to sleep. We both slept through the night.

The next night, again it worked. And I didn't really have to hold my tongue with my fingers anymore. I was able to sort of rest it between my teeth without pain and more importantly, push the back of my tongue forward.

It felt almost like I was training my tongue to jut out and forward instead of just sitting in the back of my throat. After the third night, while sitting in a pub on Lake Lucerne enjoying a beautiful day, I asked my husband if I had been snoring the night before.

He thought about it and said that he was asleep and wasn't sure but that he actually thought maybe I had been quieter than usual.

I wanted to yell "I didn't! I didn't snore!" I wanted to claim victory and shove a flag in the soil and say "Here. This place. This is where I stopped snoring forever!". But I didn't. The jury was still out.

Instead, I told him what I had learned from the Swiss version of Google, that I was a tongue snorer (that got a look) and that I was going to sleep with my tongue pulled forward. I'm pretty sure that he thought I was crazy, but he was – as always – kind and supportive.

Every night since, I have put my head down and pushed my tongue forward, resting between my teeth. I find myself playing with various positions of my tongue, but I make sure to keep the back part pushed forward. Not always sticking completely out of my mouth, but definitely not in the back of my throat as it used to be.

I've done this without incident every night since. I also have found that using a simple saline nasal spray, an over-the-counter one, into my nostrils helps keep my passages clear. I do sometimes also take a decongestant, like Claritin, just to make sure I can breathe through my nose if I'm feeling stuffed up at all.

But the big news is that my epic snoring has stopped.
I have confirmed this with my husband. And he agrees.
Yippee! ☺

7 AN ADDED BONUS

On return from our trip, I had a number of close friends ask me what I've been doing differently, saying that I look like I've been working out or that my face looks very different, particularly from the side.

On our trip, I did do a lot of walking, but I also did a lot of eating. I didn't gain or lose weight on the trip. But I saw a picture that someone took of me from the side and I saw the change in my profile too.

My jawline is slightly different.

I went into my bathroom and tried to inspect my profile. I don't have a huge double chin, but my profile has changed over the years, as they do when one hits a certain age and or has a child at 40. Don't judge.

But mine is changing, still, and seemingly for the better since Switzerland.

While in front of the mirror, I stuck out my tongue and then pulled it in and relaxed. I noticed that when I stick it out, my jawline gets more strong and crisp. When I allow my tongue to relax, I get a little lump under my chin that looks like I have a larger double chin than I do. Joy.

My take – and again, I'm not a doctor – but my perspective is that my snoring solution is also serving a second purpose. I'm training the muscles in my tongue to sit more forward on their own and as a result, my jawline is more taught and firm. I hadn't intended for this to be a benefit of what I'm doing, but I'll take it.

8 IN CONCLUSION

Not everyone is a tongue snorer, so my little trick may not work for you. But the bigger revelation for me was more about our access to information. I believe that my visit to Switzerland is responsible for my new ability to sleep without snoring. I was automatically sent to the Swiss version of Google because of where I was sitting.

Alternative information came up, meaning alternative to what I found when I used the US site. I don't think that resources in the states are deliberately hiding information from consumers. But I do think that our sales and retail mentality may be creating an information glut on the internet and that search engine optimization and sales efforts may be creating a climate where important information and helpful facts are hidden behind all the hype of what we can buy and trade.

I'm thankful to Google and to whoever posted that article I found in the middle of the night in Switzerland, when my husband woke me and said he couldn't sleep with my snoring.

I think anyone who snores might want to test their own status as a tongue snorer. Or look for more info by searching using another country's search tools. Not because ours are bad but for the fresh perspective. How can that be a bad thing?

Good luck to all who snore and those who love them. I wish you peace.

ABOUT THE AUTHOR

Julie Niehoff is a public speaker, writer and hockey mom.
She lives in Austin, Texas with 3 kids, a dog and her
Texas blues man. She works for Constant Contact as Director of
Education & Development and is a regular small business
contributor for The Huffington Post.
Julie can be found on Twitter – her handle is @JulieNiehoff.

www.ingramcontent.com/pod-product-compliance
Lightning Source LLC
Chambersburg PA
CBHW070407290526
45790CB00004B/1662